HERBAL REMEDIES FOR CIRRHOSIS:

"Nurturing Your Liver Back to Health"

Dr. Evelyn Stormhaven

Contents

INTRODUCTION

Welcome to a journey where ancient knowledge meets contemporary wellness. In a world where we're increasingly attracted to the healing powers of nature, herbal medicines provide a beacon of hope and promise, particularly for people confronting the problems of cirrhosis.

Cirrhosis, a disorder characterized by liver scarring, necessitates a comprehensive approach to healing. Herbal medicines, firmly entrenched in traditional medicine, have emerged as influential allies in the struggle against this persistent illness. Join us as we examine the age-old knowledge and current science underlying herbal medicines intended to promote liver health and increase your quality of life.

In this journey, we'll unearth the mysteries of herbs, including milk thistle, dandelion root, and turmeric, uncovering their power to calm, heal, and revitalize. Together, we'll traverse the subtleties of preparation, dosing, and mixing herbs with lifestyle modifications, providing you with a path to treating cirrhosis with the support of Mother Nature herself.

Prepare to be intrigued by the possibilities, empowered by information, and motivated to take responsibility for your health. Join us on this illuminating voyage into the realm of herbal treatments for cirrhosis, where the power of nature awaits your embrace.

CHAPTER ONE

What Is Cirrhosis?

Cirrhosis is a late stage of scarring (fibrosis) of the liver caused by long-term liver injury and inflammation. The liver, a critical organ in the body, has the astonishing capacity to regenerate and heal itself. However, when it is continually wounded over time, good liver tissue is replaced by scar tissue, leading to cirrhosis.

Here are crucial aspects concerning cirrhosis:

1. **Causes:** Cirrhosis may develop from many liver illnesses and disorders, including persistent alcoholism, hepatitis (such as hepatitis B, C, and D), fatty liver disease (non-alcoholic steatohepatitis or NASH), and other conditions that cause liver inflammation and damage.

2. **Scarring:** The liver is made up of tiny units called lobules, which are made up of liver cells (hepatocytes) that are responsible for performing vital processes, including detoxification, metabolism, and the creation of proteins. As cirrhosis advances, scar tissue grows inside the liver, altering the typical structure and function of the organ.

3. **Symptoms:** In the early stages, cirrhosis can not generate visible signs. However, as the condition

proceeds, patients may have weariness, weakness, easy bruising, jaundice (yellowing of the skin and eyes), swelling in the belly and legs (ascites and edema), disorientation, and bleeding from the gastrointestinal system.

4. **Problems:** Cirrhosis may lead to various significant issues, including portal hypertension (high blood pressure in the liver's blood veins), liver cancer, liver failure, and a heightened risk of infections.

5. **Diagnosis:** Doctors diagnose cirrhosis by a combination of medical history, physical examination, blood tests, imaging procedures (such as ultrasound or CT scans), and occasionally a liver biopsy to examine the amount of liver damage.

6. **Therapy:** The therapy of cirrhosis generally focuses on resolving the underlying cause and controlling its consequences. This may require lifestyle adjustments (such as alcohol cessation), antiviral drugs for viral hepatitis, dietary modifications, medications to control symptoms, and, in extreme situations, liver transplants.

7. **Prevention:** Cirrhosis may frequently be avoided by avoiding excessive alcohol intake, practicing safe sex to prevent hepatitis, and being vaccinated against hepatitis B. Early detection and effective medical treatment are critical in preventing cirrhosis

from developing or worsening for patients with existing liver disorders.

Cirrhosis is a severe and irreversible disorder. Thus, early identification and management are crucial to slow down its course and enhance the quality of life for individuals afflicted. Regular medical check-ups and maintaining a healthy lifestyle may play a vital role in avoiding or controlling cirrhosis.

Causes and Risk Factors

The development of cirrhosis is often connected with specific causes and risk factors that contribute to persistent liver damage and scarring. Understanding these causes and risk factors is critical for prevention and early intervention. Here are some of the fundamental causes and risk factors for cirrhosis:

1. Chronic Alcohol Abuse:
Excessive and sustained alcohol intake is one of the most prevalent causes of cirrhosis. Alcohol directly destroys liver cells, resulting in inflammation and scarring over time.

2. Chronic Viral Hepatitis:
Chronic infection with hepatitis viruses, notably hepatitis B, C, and D, may lead to cirrhosis. These viruses induce continuous inflammation and liver cell destruction.

3. Non-Alcoholic Fatty Liver Disease (NAFLD) and Non-Alcoholic Steatohepatitis (NASH):

NAFLD and NASH are conditions defined by the buildup of fat in the liver. Over time, NASH, in particular, may proceed to cirrhosis.

4. Autoimmune Liver Diseases:

Autoimmune liver illnesses, including autoimmune hepatitis, primary biliary cirrhosis, and primary sclerosing cholangitis, involve the immune system wrongly targeting the liver, causing persistent inflammation and damage.

5. Genetic Disorders:

Inherited genetic diseases such as hemochromatosis, Wilson's disease, and alpha-1 antitrypsin deficiency may alter the liver's capacity to absorb and retain certain chemicals, leading to liver damage and cirrhosis.

6. Chronic Heart Disease:

Heart disorders that cause long-term congestive heart failure may result in a backlog of blood flow into the liver, leading to congestion and cirrhosis (a disease known as cardiac cirrhosis).

7. Medications and Toxins:

Certain drugs, such as methotrexate and isoniazid, and exposure to poisons like vinyl chloride and arsenic may lead to liver damage and cirrhosis.

8. Biliary Tract Disorders:

Conditions that damage the bile ducts, such as biliary atresia, may impair the passage of bile from the liver, leading to cirrhosis.

9. Cryptogenic Cirrhosis:

In rare situations, the actual etiology of cirrhosis cannot be discovered, which is called cryptogenic cirrhosis. It may develop from undiscovered genetic, autoimmune, or viral causes.

10. Obesity and Metabolic Syndrome:

Obesity and metabolic syndrome, which includes disorders including high blood pressure, high cholesterol, and insulin resistance, might contribute to the development of NAFLD and NASH.

11. Age and Gender:

Cirrhosis may afflict persons of any age; however, it tends to be more frequent in middle-aged and older adults. Some kinds of cirrhosis, such as primary biliary cirrhosis, are more frequent in women.

12. Ethnicity and Geographic Location:

The frequency of various liver disorders and cirrhosis might vary by ethnicity and geographical location owing to changes in hepatitis prevalence and genetic variables.

It's crucial to understand that cirrhosis may develop slowly over many years, and people may not have visible symptoms until the condition is severe. Early diagnosis via medical check-ups and addressing risk factors is crucial to avoiding or treating cirrhosis successfully. Lifestyle adjustments, immunization against hepatitis, and effective medical treatment for underlying illnesses may dramatically lower the incidence of cirrhosis.

Symptoms and Diagnosis

Cirrhosis is a disorder that may develop gradually, and patients may not have visible symptoms in its early stages. However, various symptoms might appear when the illness advances, and liver function is reduced. Additionally, cirrhosis may be identified by numerous medical tests and exams. Here's an outline of the signs and diagnostic techniques connected with cirrhosis:

Symptoms of Cirrhosis:

1. **Weariness:** Chronic weariness and weakness are typical in patients with cirrhosis owing to the reduced liver's capacity to process and store energy.

2. **Jaundice:** Yellowing of the skin and the whites of the eyes (jaundice) is a typical symptom of liver disease. It happens when bilirubin, a yellow pigment, builds up in the body.

3. **Abdominal Swelling (Ascites):** Cirrhosis may lead to fluid buildup in the abdominal cavity, leading to abdominal swelling and pain.

4. **Leg Swelling (Edema):** Fluid retention may also cause swelling in the legs and ankles.

5. **Bruising and Easy Bleeding:** A damaged liver may generate fewer clotting factors, leading to easy bruising and a heightened risk of bleeding.

6. **Itchy Skin:** The accumulation of toxins in the bloodstream may contribute to itching and skin rashes.

7. **Dark Urine and Pale Stools:** Changes in the color of urine (darker) and stools (paler) may develop owing to liver failure.

8. **Loss of Appetite and Weight Loss:** Digestive disorders and diminished appetite might contribute to accidental weight loss.

9. **Confusion and Cognitive alterations:** In advanced cirrhosis, a condition known as hepatic encephalopathy may arise, producing mess, forgetfulness, and changes in cognitive function.

10. **Spider-Like Blood Vessels (Spider Angiomas):** Small, red spider-like blood vessels may form on the skin.

11. **Nausea and Vomiting:** Digestive symptoms might develop, including nausea and vomiting.

1. **Medical History and Physical Examination:** A doctor will take a complete medical history and physical examination to identify symptoms, risk factors, and evidence of cirrhosis.

2. **Blood Tests:** Blood tests may show liver function, including levels of liver enzymes, bilirubin, and clotting factors. Elevated levels of liver enzymes and bilirubin are typical in cirrhosis.

3. **Imaging Studies:** Ultrasound, CT scans, and MRI scans may offer pictures of the liver, helping to estimate its size and discover symptoms of cirrhosis, such as nodules or scarring.

4. **FibroScan or Transient Elastography:** This non-invasive test assesses liver stiffness, which might be symptomatic of cirrhosis.

5. **Liver Biopsy:** In certain circumstances, a liver biopsy may be done to collect a tiny tissue sample for microscopic inspection. This may assist in establishing the level of liver damage and pinpoint the underlying cause of cirrhosis.

6. **Endoscopy:** In situations of suspected varices (enlarged blood vessels in the esophagus or stomach), an endoscopy may be done to see these veins and evaluate the risk of bleeding.

7. **Ascitic Fluid Analysis:** A fluid sample may be removed and examined to discover its etiology if ascites are present.

8. **Other Tests:** Additional tests may be conducted to check particular areas of liver function and uncover underlying reasons, such as viral hepatitis serology or autoimmune markers.

Diagnosing cirrhosis often includes a mix of these procedures, since the illness may have multiple underlying causes and manifest with various symptoms. Early identification is critical for treating cirrhosis efficiently and avoiding additional liver damage. Once diagnosed, effective therapy and lifestyle adjustments may help delay the course of the illness and enhance the patient's quality of life.

Stages of Cirrhosis

Cirrhosis is a progressive liver condition characterized by the scarring (fibrosis) of liver tissue over time. The severity of cirrhosis is sometimes divided into stages or grades to assist healthcare personnel in identifying the level of liver damage and guide treatment options. Several techniques are used to classify the stages of cirrhosis, but one prominent way is the Child-Pugh score and the Model for End-Stage Liver Disease (MELD) score. Here's a summary of the phases of cirrhosis using the Child-Pugh classification:

The Child-Pugh classification system provides points to five clinical parameters linked to liver function:

1. **Total Bilirubin Levels:** Measures bilirubin, a waste product that may build in the circulation when the liver is damaged.

2. **Serum Albumin Levels:** Reflects the liver's capacity to make proteins, including albumin.

3. **Prothrombin Time (INR):** Evaluates blood clotting time, which may be extended in cirrhosis owing to lower synthesis of clotting factors.

4. **Ascites:** Presence of abdominal fluid buildup (ascites), a symptom of severe liver disease.

5. **Hepatic Encephalopathy:** The existence and severity of cognitive abnormalities and confusion owing to liver malfunction.

Based on the ratings given to these factors, patients with cirrhosis are divided into three Child-Pugh stages:

- **Child-Pugh Class A:** This stage suggests less severe cirrhosis with a reasonably favorable prognosis. It is defined by a total score of 5 to 6 points.

- **Child-Pugh Class B:** In this stage, cirrhosis is considered moderately severe, with a total score of 7 to 9 points. The outlook is worse than Class A.

- **Child-Pugh Class C:** This stage shows severe cirrhosis with a score of 10 or more points. It has a worse prognosis and is connected with a greater risk of complications.

Model for End-Stage Liver Disease (MELD) Score:

In addition to Child-Pugh, the MELD score is utilized for selecting individuals for liver transplantation and measuring the severity of liver disease. The MELD score is derived from three laboratory values: serum bilirubin, serum creatinine, and the INR. It produces a numerical score corresponding with the risk of death due to liver disease.

The MELD score ranges from 6 to 40, with higher values indicating more severe illness. Patients with higher MELD scores are often considered for liver transplantation.

It's vital to remember that the staging and categorization of cirrhosis are used to guide treatment choices, predict outcomes, and prioritize individuals for transplantation. Cirrhosis is a progressive disorder, and people may advance from one stage to another over time, mainly if the underlying source of liver damage is not appropriately addressed. Regular monitoring and medical treatment are necessary for controlling cirrhosis and avoiding complications.

CHAPTER TWO

The Role of Herbal Remedies

Why Consider Herbal Remedies?

Considering herbal therapies for different health disorders, including cirrhosis, is a decision that some persons make for numerous reasons. It's vital to approach herbal medicines cautiously and with a healthcare expert since their efficacy and safety might vary. Here are some reasons why individuals may explore herbal therapies for cirrhosis:

1. **Potential Symptom Relief:** Herbal medicines may relieve some symptoms linked with cirrhosis, such as weariness, stomach pain, and itching. Some plants are considered to contain qualities that may treat particular illnesses.

2. **Complementary Therapy:** Herbal medicines are occasionally used in combination with standard medical treatments as complementary therapy. They may be a means to increase traditional therapies' efficacy or control adverse effects.

3. **Seen Natural and Holistic Approach:** Many individuals are attracted to herbal medicines because they are seen as natural and holistic. Some folks prefer these solutions since they feel less likely to induce adverse effects or damage the body.

4. **Cultural & Traditional Use:** Herbal treatments have been utilized in numerous cultures for ages to address various health conditions. People from countries with significant traditional herbal medicine traditions may resort to these therapies owing to cultural beliefs and familiarity.

5. **Potential Liver Support:** Certain herbs are known to have hepatoprotective characteristics, meaning they may help protect the liver from further harm. This might be intriguing to persons with cirrhosis since maintaining liver function is a crucial therapy objective.

6. **Personal Experience or Anecdotal Evidence:** Some persons may have had good experiences with herbal treatments or know of others who have benefitted from them. Anecdotal evidence may affect people's choices to seek herbal remedies.

7. **Restricted Conventional therapy choices:** In certain situations, cirrhosis may reach an advanced stage when conventional therapy choices are limited, and a person may seek alternative treatments, including herbal therapies, as a last resort.

It's crucial to pursue herbal therapies for cirrhosis with prudence and educated decision-making:

- **Consultation with Healthcare Providers:** Before commencing any herbal therapy, speaking with a healthcare professional, ideally one with knowledge in both conventional and alternative medicine, is vital. They may give recommendations on the safety and suitability of various herbal treatments.

- **Safety Considerations:** Not all herbal therapies are safe or acceptable for everyone, particularly for persons with cirrhosis, since the liver's capacity to process chemicals may be hampered. Some herbs may interfere with drugs or cause liver disease.

- **Quality and Standardization:** The quality and purity of herbal items vary considerably. Look for trustworthy producers and goods that comply with quality and safety regulations.

- **Monitoring and Follow-up:** If herbal medicines are taken with conventional therapies, frequent monitoring and follow-up with a healthcare professional are needed to evaluate their efficacy and ensure no harmful interactions occur.

While herbal therapies have the potential to give advantages, they should be incorporated into a complete treatment strategy that includes lifestyle modifications, conventional medical care, and continuing monitoring to successfully manage cirrhosis and associated consequences.

Safety and Precautions

Safety and precautions are of crucial significance while contemplating herbal medicines, particularly for persons with cirrhosis or other underlying health issues. While herbal medicines have potential advantages, they can also bring hazards, interact with drugs, or worsen specific health concerns. Here are some crucial safety factors and measures to bear in mind while utilizing herbal therapies for cirrhosis:

Consultation with a Healthcare Provider:

Before starting any herbal treatment, always contact a healthcare physician, ideally educated in herbal therapy and liver health. They can analyze your unique health situation, prescribe proper medicines, and track your progress.

1. Transparency About Herbal Use:
Inform your healthcare physician about herbal treatments, supplements, or complementary therapies since they may interfere with drugs or impact your liver function.

2. Herb-Drug Interactions:
Some plants may interact with prescription and over-the-counter drugs, possibly lowering their efficacy or producing bad effects. Common medicines used by persons with cirrhosis, such as diuretics or blood-thinning medications, may interact with herbs. Your healthcare practitioner may advise on possible interactions.

3. Liver Function Assessment:

Individuals with cirrhosis should undergo frequent liver function examinations, including testing for liver enzymes, bilirubin levels, and clotting factors. Herbal medicines should not affect liver function or create more liver damage.

4. Quality and Safety of Herbal Products:

Choose herbal goods from recognized suppliers that conform to quality and safety regulations. Look for items branded with the United States Pharmacopeia (USP) or other quality certifications.

5. Dosage & Administration:

Follow the prescribed dose and administration instructions specified on the herbal product's package or as suggested by your healthcare practitioner. Do not exceed the recommended dosage.

6. Monitoring for Adverse Effects:

When utilizing herbal therapies, pay particular attention to any side effects or strange symptoms. If you encounter any harmful effects, cease usage and inform your healthcare professional.

7. Potential Allergies or Sensitivities:

Be careful of any allergies or sensitivities you may have to certain plants. Cross-check the contents of herbal goods to prevent possible allergies.

8. Liver-Toxic Herbs:

Some herbs may be harmful to the liver and may aggravate cirrhosis. Avoid plants connected with liver damage, including comfrey, kava, and chaparral.

9. Individualized Approach:

Herbal therapies should be selected depending on your unique health demands and the underlying reasons for cirrhosis. What works for one person may only work for one person. Therefore, tailored treatment strategies are vital.

10. Herbal Preparation Methods:

Some herbal medicines are accessible in various forms, such as capsules, tinctures, teas, or extracts. Consider which shape is most suited for you and follow the correct preparation and storage requirements.

11. Regular Follow-Up:

Maintain frequent follow-up consultations with your healthcare practitioner to review the efficiency of herbal treatments, check liver function, and alter therapy as required.

Remember that herbal therapies do not replace conventional medical treatment in controlling cirrhosis. They should be included in a complete therapy strategy for lifestyle adjustments and other medical procedures. Always emphasize safety and seek expert counsel while taking herbal therapies, particularly if you have a previous liver problem like cirrhosis.

Herbal Remedies vs. Conventional Treatments

The choice between herbal therapies and conventional treatments for cirrhosis is an essential decision that should be made in cooperation with a healthcare expert. Each technique has its benefits and concerns, and the usefulness of one over the other may depend on individual circumstances, the severity of cirrhosis, and the underlying reasons. Here's a comparison of herbal therapies and conventional treatments for cirrhosis:

Herbal Remedies:

Advantages:

1. **Perceived Natural Approach:** Herbal medicines are taken from natural sources, such as plants and herbs, which some individuals find attractive since they may assume they are less likely to create unwanted effects.

2. **Potential Symptom Relief:** Certain herbs may relieve specific cirrhosis-related symptoms, such as weariness, stomach pain, or itching.

3. **Complimentary Therapy:** Herbal medicines may be used with conventional therapies as positive therapy to address particular symptoms or promote general well-being.

4. **Cultural & Traditional Use:** In certain societies, traditional herbal medical techniques have been handed down for centuries, and people may have a deep cultural connection to these medicines.

Considerations:

1. **Limited Scientific Evidence:** Many herbal medicines need more thorough scientific trials to validate their safety and effectiveness for cirrhosis. The efficacy of herbal remedies might vary greatly.

2. **Potential Interactions:** Some plants may interact with drugs or other herbs, possibly altering their efficacy or producing harmful effects.

3. **Safety Concerns:** Certain herbs may be hazardous to the liver and should be avoided, particularly by those with cirrhosis. Proper dosage and safety measures are needed.

4. **Lack of Standardization:** Herbal products might vary in quality, potency, and purity. Choosing reliable manufacturers and goods is vital.

Advantages:

1. **Proof-Based:** Conventional therapies for cirrhosis are based on scientific research and clinical studies, offering better proof of their safety and efficacy.

2. **Well-created Protocols:** Healthcare experts have created treatment protocols for cirrhosis, including drugs, lifestyle guidelines, and medical treatments like liver transplantation.

3. **Monitoring and competence:** Conventional therapies entail frequent liver function and disease development monitoring by healthcare experts with competence in liver care.

4. **Approved medicines:** Some medicines used in traditional therapy, such as antiviral treatments for viral hepatitis or pharmaceuticals to control problems, have been approved by regulatory bodies and have a documented track record.

Considerations:

1. **Potential Side Effects:** Conventional drugs for cirrhosis may have side effects, and some may need close monitoring and control.

2. **Not a Cure:** Conventional therapies may slow the advancement of cirrhosis and control symptoms but may not cure the underlying liver illness.

3. **Cost:** Some traditional treatments and medical operations, such as liver transplantation, may be pricey.

In many circumstances, a mix of both techniques may be explored. Healthcare experts may propose conventional therapies to address the underlying causes of cirrhosis and manage complications while adding specialized herbal medicines for symptom alleviation or as supplemental therapy. People with cirrhosis must have open and honest talks with their healthcare professionals, reveal their use of herbal treatments, and work together to build a complete treatment plan that promotes safety and efficacy.

CHAPTER THREE

Herbal Remedies for Liver Health

Milk Thistle with Silymarin

Milk thistle (Silybum marianum) and its active ingredient, silymarin, are commonly studied for their possible advantages in maintaining liver health, especially in liver diseases like cirrhosis. Here are various methods to make and utilize milk thistle and silymarin for cirrhosis health:

1. Milk Thistle Extract or Supplements:

- **Milk Thistle Capsules or Tablets:** Commercially accessible milk thistle supplements frequently come in capsule or tablet form. Follow the prescribed dose guidelines on the product label or as your healthcare practitioner suggests. Quality and potency might vary, so select a recognized brand.

- **Liquid Extract:** Milk thistle extracts in liquid form are also available. These may be combined with water or juice and consumed according to the prescribed dose.

Ingredients:

- One teaspoon of crushed milk thistle seeds (you may purchase them at health food shops or online)
- 1 cup of hot water

Directions:
1. Crush the milk thistle seeds using a mortar and pestle.
2. Place the smashed seeds in a cup.
3. Pour boiling water over the seeds.
4. Cover the cup and let it steep for 10-15 minutes.
5. Strain the tea to remove the seeds.
6. Drink the tea while it's still warm.
7. Frequency: You may eat milk thistle tea once or twice a day.

Ingredients:
- Dried milk thistle seeds
- High-proof alcohol (such as vodka or brandy)

Directions:
1. Place dried milk thistle seeds in a glass container.
2. Cover the seeds fully with the high-proof alcohol.
3. Seal the jar securely.
4. Store the jar in a cold, dark area for approximately 4-6 weeks, stirring it gently every few days.

5. After steeping, strain the liquid through a fine-mesh strainer or cheesecloth to remove the seeds.
6. Transfer the tincture to a dark glass bottle for storage.
7. **Usage:** Take a few drops of the tincture (usually 20-30 drops) mixed with water, as a healthcare provider recommends.

4. Considerations:

- **Consult a Healthcare Provider:** Before using milk thistle or silymarin supplements, tea, or tinctures for cirrhosis or any other health condition, it's crucial to consult your healthcare provider. They can assess your specific situation, provide guidance on dosages, and ensure there are no contraindications or interactions with medications you may be taking.

- **Assess Progress:** Regularly evaluate your liver function and general health while utilizing milk thistle or silymarin. Discuss any changes in your condition with your healthcare professional.

- **Safety:** While milk thistle is usually considered safe, it may induce moderate gastrointestinal issues in some persons. Allergic reactions are rare but possible. If you encounter any ill effects, cease usage and seek medical assistance.

Dandelion Root

Dandelion root (Taraxacum officinale) is another herbal remedy that is sometimes considered for its potential benefits in supporting liver health, including in cases of cirrhosis. It can be prepared in various ways, such as dandelion root tea or tincture. Here's how to prepare and use dandelion root for cirrhosis health:

Dandelion Root Tea:

Ingredients:
- Dried dandelion root (readily available in health food stores or online)
- Hot water

Directions:
1. Measure 1-2 tablespoons of dried dandelion root per cup of boiling water.
2. Boil the water over the dried dandelion root in a teapot or cup.
3. Cover the container and let it steep for about 10-15 minutes.
4. Strain the tea to remove the dandelion root pieces.
5. You can add honey or lemon for flavor if desired.
6. Drink the tea while it's still warm.
7. Frequency: You can consume dandelion root tea up to 2-3 times a day or as a healthcare provider recommends.

Ingredients:

- Fresh dandelion roots or dried dandelion root (chopped)
- High-proof alcohol (e.g., vodka or brandy)

Directions:

1. If using fresh dandelion roots, wash and chop them into small pieces. If using dried dandelion root, you may omit this step.
2. Place the chopped dandelion root in a glass container.
3. Cover the root fully with the high-proof alcohol.
4. Seal the jar securely.
5. Store the jar in a cold, dark area for approximately 4-6 weeks, stirring it gently every few days.
6. After steeping, strain the liquid through a fine-mesh strainer or cheesecloth to remove the root bits.
7. Transfer the tincture to a dark glass container for storage.
8. **Usage:** Take a few drops of the dandelion root tincture (usually 20-30 drops) combined with water, as a healthcare practitioner prescribes.

Considerations:

- **Visit a Healthcare practitioner:** Before taking dandelion root preparations for cirrhosis or any other health problem, visiting your healthcare practitioner is vital. They may examine your unique health status, give recommendations on doses, and verify that there are no contraindications or conflicts with drugs you may be taking.

- **Assess Progress:** Regularly assess your liver function and general health using dandelion root. Discuss any changes in your condition with your healthcare professional.

- **Safety:** Dandelion root is usually considered safe for most individuals, whether taken as a dietary supplement or herbal treatment. However, it may produce moderate gastrointestinal issues in some persons. Allergic responses are infrequent but possible. If you encounter any ill effects, cease usage and seek medical assistance.

Turmeric and Curcumin

Turmeric (Curcuma longa) and its main ingredient, curcumin, are renowned for their potential anti-inflammatory and antioxidant qualities, which may aid persons with cirrhosis. Turmeric may be prepared in numerous ways to integrate it into your diet. Here's how to make and utilize turmeric and curcumin for cirrhosis health:

Ingredients:
- Turmeric powder (readily accessible at grocery shops or online)
- Hot water, milk, or other liquids

Directions:
1. Add ½ to 1 teaspoon of turmeric powder to a cup.
2. Boil water, milk, or any beverage of your choosing.
3. Pour the heated liquid over the turmeric powder.
4. Stir vigorously to dissolve the turmeric.
5. You may add honey, ginger, or black pepper for taste and improved absorption of curcumin.
6. Drink the turmeric-infused beverage while it's still warm.
7. **Frequency:** You may eat turmeric-infused beverages once or twice a day.

Ingredients:
- Turmeric capsules or pills (available at health food shops or online)
- Water

Directions:
1. Follow the prescribed dose guidelines on the product label or as your healthcare practitioner suggests.

2. Take the turmeric capsules or pills with water or as instructed.
3. Frequency: Follow the prescribed dose on the product label or your healthcare provider's recommendations.

3. Turmeric and Curcumin Extracts:

Ingredients:

- Turmeric or curcumin extracts in liquid or pill form

Directions:

1. Follow the recommended dose guidelines indicated on the product label or as suggested by your healthcare practitioner.
2. **Frequency:** Follow the prescribed dose on the product label or your healthcare provider's recommendations.

Considerations:

- **See a Healthcare practitioner:** Before taking turmeric or curcumin supplements or adding turmeric to your diet for cirrhosis or any other health problem, it's crucial to see your healthcare practitioner. They may examine your unique health status, give recommendations on doses, and verify that there are no contraindications or conflicts with drugs you may be taking.

- **Black Pepper:** Combining turmeric with black pepper (which includes piperine) helps improve the absorption of curcumin. Consider adding a sprinkle of black pepper while ingesting turmeric.

- **Assess Progress:** Regularly assess your liver function and general health using turmeric or curcumin. Discuss any changes in your condition with your healthcare professional.

- **Safety:** Turmeric and curcumin are usually considered safe when ingested at dietary levels. However, large dosages or long-term usage of supplements may have possible adverse effects or interactions with drugs. Follow appropriate doses and instructions.

Turmeric and curcumin may be a significant element of a comprehensive approach to maintaining liver function in instances of cirrhosis.

Schisandra Berry

Schisandra berries (Schisandra chinensis) are recognized for their possible hepatoprotective qualities and may be considered in maintaining liver health, notably in instances of cirrhosis. Schisandra berries may be made as a tea or tincture. Here's how to prepare and utilize Schisandra berries for cirrhosis health:

Schisandra Berry Tea:

Ingredients:
- Dried Schisandra berries (available at health food shops or online)
- Hot water

Directions:
1. Measure 1-2 tablespoons of dried Schisandra berries per cup of boiling water.
2. Boil the water over the dried Schisandra berries in a teapot or cup.
3. Cover the container and let it soak for approximately 10-15 minutes.
4. Strain the tea to remove the Schisandra berries.
5. You may add honey or lemon for taste if preferred.
6. Drink the tea while it's still warm.
7. **Frequency:** You may eat Schisandra berry tea up to 2-3 times a day or as directed by a healthcare expert.

Schisandra Berry Tincture:

Ingredients:
- Dried Schisandra berries
- High-proof alcohol (e.g., vodka or brandy)

Directions:
1. Place dried Schisandra berries in a glass container.
2. Cover the fruit fully with the high-proof alcohol.
3. Seal the jar securely.

4. Store the jar in a cold, dark area for approximately 4-6 weeks, stirring it gently every few days.
5. After steeping, strain the liquid through a fine-mesh strainer or cheesecloth to remove the berries.
6. Transfer the tincture to a dark glass container for storage.
7. **Usage:** Take a few drops of the Schisandra berry tincture (usually 20-30 drops) combined with water, as a healthcare expert prescribes.

Considerations:

- **Visit a Healthcare practitioner:** Before consuming Schisandra berries or Schisandra berry preparations for cirrhosis or any other health issue, visit your healthcare practitioner. They may examine your unique health status, give recommendations on doses, and verify that there are no contraindications or conflicts with drugs you may be taking.

- **Assess Progress:** Regularly assess your liver function and general health while consuming Schisandra berries. Discuss any changes in your condition with your healthcare professional.

- **Safety:** Schisandra berries are usually considered safe for most individuals when ingested in dietary proportions. However, large dosages or long-term usage of supplements may have possible negative effects or interactions with drugs. Follow appropriate doses and instructions.

Schisandra berries may be a component of a comprehensive strategy for promoting liver health in instances of cirrhosis. However, they should not replace traditional medical therapy and should be taken with prescription drugs and medical supervision. Always prioritize safety and cooperate with your healthcare physician to build a complete treatment plan.

CHAPTER FOUR

Detoxifying Herbs

Burdock Root

Burdock root (Arctium lappa) is another herbal treatment that is occasionally investigated for its possible advantages in maintaining liver function, notably in instances of cirrhosis. Burdock root may be prepared in numerous ways, such as burdock root tea or tincture. Here's how to prepare and utilize burdock root for cirrhosis health:

Burdock Root Tea:

Ingredients:
- Dried burdock root (readily accessible at health food shops or online)
- Hot water

Directions:
1. Measure roughly 1-2 tablespoons of dried burdock root per cup of boiling water.
2. Boil the water over the dried burdock root in a teapot or cup.
3. Cover the container and let it soak for approximately 10-15 minutes.
4. Strain the tea to remove the burdock root bits.
5. You may add honey or lemon for taste if preferred.
6. Drink the burdock root tea while it's still warm.

7. **Frequency:** You may take burdock root tea up to 2-3 times daily or as directed by a healthcare expert.

Burdock Root Tincture:

Ingredients:

- Dried burdock root (chopped)
- High-proof alcohol (e.g., vodka or brandy)

Directions:

1. Place dried burdock root in a glass container.
2. Cover the root fully with the high-proof alcohol.
3. Seal the jar securely.
4. Store the jar in a cold, dark area for approximately 4-6 weeks, stirring it gently every few days.
5. After steeping, strain the liquid through a fine-mesh strainer or cheesecloth to remove the root bits.
6. Transfer the tincture to a dark glass container for storage.
7. **Usage:** Take a few drops of the burdock root tincture (usually 20-30 drops) combined with water, as a healthcare expert prescribes.

Considerations:

- **Visit a Healthcare practitioner:** Before using burdock root or burdock root products for cirrhosis or any other health problem, visit your healthcare practitioner. They may examine your unique health status, give recommendations on doses, and verify that there are no contraindications or conflicts with drugs you may be taking.

- **Assess Progress:** Regularly assess your liver function and general health using burdock root. Discuss any changes in your condition with your healthcare professional.

- **Safety:** Burdock root is usually considered safe when ingested at dietary levels. However, large dosages or long-term usage of supplements may have possible adverse effects or interactions with drugs. Follow appropriate doses and instructions.

Burdock root may be a component of a comprehensive strategy for promoting liver health in cirrhosis. However, it should not replace traditional medical therapy and should be taken with prescription drugs and medical supervision. Always prioritize safety and cooperate with your healthcare physician to build a complete treatment plan.

Artichoke Leaf

Artichoke leaf (Cynara scolymus) is another herbal medicine occasionally investigated for its possible advantages in maintaining liver function, notably in cirrhosis. Artichoke leaf may be prepared in numerous ways, such as tea or leaf extract. Here's how to prepare and utilize artichoke leaf for cirrhosis health:

Artichoke Leaf Tea:

Ingredients:

- Dried artichoke leaves (readily accessible at health food shops or online)
- Hot water

Directions:

1. Measure approximately 1-2 teaspoons of dried artichoke leaves per cup of hot water.
2. Boil the water over the dried artichoke leaves in a teapot or cup.
3. Cover the container and let it soak for approximately 10-15 minutes.
4. Strain the tea to remove the artichoke leaf pieces.
5. You may add honey or lemon for taste if preferred.
6. Drink the artichoke leaf tea while it's still warm.
7. **Frequency:** You can consume artichoke leaf tea up to 2-3 times a day or as a healthcare provider recommends.

Artichoke Leaf Extract or Capsules:

Ingredients:

- Artichoke leaf extract or capsules (available in health food stores or online)
- Water

Directions:

1. Follow the prescribed dose guidelines on the product label or as your healthcare practitioner suggests.
2. Take the artichoke leaf extract or capsules with a glass of water or as directed.
3. **Frequency:** Follow the prescribed dose on the product label or your healthcare provider's recommendations.

Considerations:

- **Consult a Healthcare Provider:** Before using artichoke leaf or artichoke leaf preparations for cirrhosis or any other health condition, consult your healthcare provider. They may examine your unique health status, give recommendations on doses, and verify that there are no contraindications or conflicts with drugs you may be taking.

- **Monitor Progress:** Use artichoke leaf to monitor your liver function and overall health. Discuss any changes in your condition with your healthcare professional.

- **Safety:** Artichoke leaf is generally considered safe for most people when consumed in dietary amounts. However, large dosages or long-term usage of supplements may have possible adverse effects or interactions with drugs. Follow appropriate doses and instructions.

Artichoke leaf can be a part of a holistic approach to supporting liver health in cases of cirrhosis. However, it should not replace traditional medical therapy and should be taken with prescription drugs and medical supervision. Always prioritize safety and cooperate with your healthcare physician to build a complete treatment plan.

Yellow Dock

Yellow dock (Rumex crispus) is a herb traditionally used for various medicinal purposes, including supporting liver health. It's known for its potential detoxifying properties and may be considered in cases of cirrhosis or other liver-related conditions. Yellow dock can be prepared in various forms, such as yellow dock tea or yellow dock tincture. Here's how to prepare and use yellow dock for cirrhosis health:

Yellow Dock Tea:

Ingredients:
- Dried yellow dock root (readily available in health food stores or online)
- Hot water

Directions:
1. Measure approximately 1-2 teaspoons of dried yellow dock root per cup of hot water.
2. Boil the water and pour it over the dried yellow dock root in a teapot or cup.

3. Cover the container and let it soak for approximately 10-15 minutes.
4. Strain the tea to remove the yellow dock root fragments.
5. You may add honey or lemon for taste if preferred.
6. Drink the yellow dock tea while it's still warm.
7. **Frequency:** You may have yellow dock tea up to 2-3 times a day or as a healthcare expert prescribes.

Yellow Dock Tincture:

Ingredients:

- Dried yellow dock root (chopped)
- High-proof alcohol (e.g., vodka or brandy)

Directions:

1. Place dried yellow dock root in a glass container.
2. Cover the root fully with the high-proof alcohol.
3. Seal the jar securely.
4. Store the jar in a cold, dark area for approximately 4-6 weeks, stirring it gently every few days.
5. After steeping, strain the liquid through a fine-mesh strainer or cheesecloth to remove the root bits.
6. Transfer the tincture to a dark glass container for storage.
7. **Usage:** Take a few drops of the yellow dock tincture (usually 20-30 drops) combined with water, as a healthcare practitioner prescribes.

Considerations:

- **Visit a Healthcare practitioner:** Before using yellow dock or yellow dock preparations for cirrhosis or any other health problem, visit your healthcare practitioner. They may examine your unique health status, give recommendations on doses, and verify that there are no contraindications or conflicts with drugs you may be taking.

- **Assess Progress:** Regularly assess your liver function and general health while taking Yellow Dock. Discuss any changes in your condition with your healthcare professional.

- **Safety:** Yellow dock is usually considered safe when ingested at dietary levels. However, large dosages or long-term usage of supplements may have possible adverse effects or interactions with drugs. Follow appropriate doses and instructions.

Yellow dock may be a component of a comprehensive strategy to promote liver health in cirrhosis. However, it should not replace traditional medical therapy and should be taken with prescription drugs and medical supervision. Always prioritize safety and cooperate with your healthcare physician to build a complete treatment plan.

Herbal Tea Blends for Detoxification

Detoxification herbal tea blends are generally produced from various herbs and botanicals renowned for their potential detoxifying and cleaning qualities. These teas help boost the body's natural cleansing processes and enhance general well-being. Here's a simple herbal tea combination for detoxification that you may try:

Detox Herbal Tea Blend:

Ingredients:

- **1 part Dandelion Root:** Dandelion root is recognized for its diuretic qualities and may help maintain liver and kidney function.

- **1 part Burdock Root:** Burdock root is supposed to assist in cleaning the blood and maintaining liver function.

- **1 part Milk Thistle Seeds:** Milk thistle is recognized for its hepatoprotective characteristics and may help protect and strengthen the liver.

- **One part Peppermint Leaves:** Peppermint gives a pleasant taste and may assist digestion.

Directions:

1. Mix equal portions of dried dandelion root, burdock root, milk thistle seeds, and peppermint leaves in a basin.

2. Use around 1-2 tablespoons of the herbal combination for a single cup of tea.

3. Boil water over the herbal combination in a teapot or cup.

4. Cover the container and let it soak for approximately 10-15 minutes.

5. Strain the tea to remove the herbal bits.

6. You may add a little honey or lemon for taste if desired.

7. Drink the detox herbal tea while it's still warm.

Frequency: You may drink this detox herbal tea mix once daily as a cleansing regimen. However, talk with a healthcare expert before beginning any detox program, particularly if you have underlying health concerns or are using drugs.

Considerations:

- **Please consult with a Healthcare practitioner:** Before beginning any detox program or utilizing detoxifying herbal teas, it's necessary to consult with a healthcare practitioner. They can give direction and guarantee that a detoxification strategy is safe and suited for your unique requirements.

- **Hydration:** Staying appropriately hydrated is vital during detoxification. Drink lots of water throughout the day in addition to herbal teas.

- **Balance:** Detoxification should be part of a balanced and healthy lifestyle that includes a good diet, frequent physical exercise, and other self-care routines.

- **Listen to Your Body:** Pay attention to how your body reacts to detoxification techniques. If you suffer unpleasant effects, cease the program and seek medical guidance.

- **Quality Herbs:** Ensure you use high-quality, organic herbs for your detox tea mix to reduce exposure to pesticides and pollutants.

Detoxification herbal teas may be a pleasant addition to your wellness regimen when taken carefully and as part of a more comprehensive plan for sustaining health and well-being.

CHAPTER FIVE

Herbal Support for Digestion

Ginger Root

Ginger root (Zingiber officinale) is a popular plant for its possible health advantages, including anti-inflammatory and digestive characteristics. While ginger root may not directly cure cirrhosis, it may help control some of the symptoms of liver disorders and improve general health. Here's how to prepare and utilize ginger root for cirrhosis health:

Ginger Root Tea:

Ingredients:
- Fresh ginger root (approximately 1-inch piece, peeled and sliced) or dried ginger (1-2 tablespoons)
- Hot water
- Honey or lemon (optional)

Directions:
1. For fresh ginger root: Peel and finely slice a 1-inch piece of ginger.

2. For dried ginger: Measure 1-2 tablespoons of dried ginger.

3. Boil water and pour it over the fresh or dried ginger in a teapot or cup.

4. Cover the container and let it soak for approximately 5-10 minutes.

5. If desired, add honey or lemon for taste.

6. Drink the ginger tea while it's still warm.

7. **Frequency:**You may eat ginger tea up to 2-3 times a day. Adjust the frequency to your liking and how well your body reacts.

Ginger Infusion:

Ingredients:
- Fresh ginger root (approximately 1-inch piece, peeled and sliced)
- Water

Directions:
1. Peel and finely slice a 1-inch piece of fresh ginger root.

2. Boil water in a pot and add the ginger slices.

3. Let the ginger simmer in the water for around 10-15 minutes.

4. Remove the pot from the heat and drain the ginger infusion into a cup.

5. Allow it to cool somewhat before drinking.

6. **Frequency:** You may eat ginger infusion once a day.

Considerations:
- **Visit a Healthcare practitioner:** Before using ginger for cirrhosis or any other health problem, it's crucial to visit your healthcare practitioner, particularly if you have liver disorders or are using drugs. Ginger may interact with some medicines or aggravate particular health issues.

- **Monitor Progress:** Pay attention to how your body reacts to ginger. Ginger is typically safe for most people when ingested in modest doses, but some individuals may develop stomach pain or other adverse effects.

- **Safety:** Avoid taking excessive amounts of ginger since it may induce heartburn, digestive difficulties, or harm medicines. Stick to modest consumption.

- **Variety:** You may alter the intensity of your ginger tea or infusion by varying the quantity of ginger used or the steeping time.

Peppermint

Peppermint (Mentha × piperita) is a plant noted for its refreshing taste and possible health advantages, including improving digestion and relieving stomach distress. While peppermint may not directly cure cirrhosis, it may help control some of the symptoms linked with liver diseases and promote overall digestive health. Here's how to make and utilize peppermint for cirrhosis health:

Peppermint Tea:

Ingredients:
- Dried peppermint leaves (readily accessible at health food shops or online)
- Hot water Honey (optional)

Directions:
1. Measure roughly 1-2 tablespoons of dried peppermint leaves per cup of hot water.

2. Boil water over the dried peppermint leaves in a teapot or cup.

3. Cover the container and let it soak for approximately 5-10 minutes.

4. If desired, add honey for taste.

5. Drink the peppermint tea while it's still warm.

6. **Frequency:**You may have peppermint tea numerous times a day, as required. Adjust the frequency to your liking and how well your body reacts.

Ingredients:
- Fresh peppermint leaves (a handful)
- Water

Directions:
1. Wash a handful of fresh peppermint leaves.

2. Boil water in a pot and add the fresh peppermint leaves.

3. Let the peppermint leaves simmer in the water for around 5-10 minutes.

4. Remove the skillet from the heat and drain the peppermint infusion into a cup.

5. Allow it to cool somewhat before drinking.

6. **Frequency:** You may sip peppermint infusion once daily or as required for digestive ease.

Considerations:

- **Visit a Healthcare practitioner:** Before using peppermint for cirrhosis or any other health problem, visit your healthcare practitioner, particularly if you have liver disorders or are taking drugs. Peppermint may interfere with some medicines or aggravate particular health issues.

- **Monitor Progress:** Pay attention to how your body reacts to peppermint. Peppermint is typically safe for most people when ingested in modest doses, although some individuals may develop stomach discomfort or other adverse effects.

- **Safety:** Peppermint is usually well-tolerated, although excessive use may induce heartburn or stomach Difficulties in specific individuals. Stick to modest consumption.

- **Variety:** You may change the intensity of your peppermint tea or infusion by adjusting the quantity of peppermint used or the steeping time.

Peppermint is a relaxing and valuable addition to your diet, particularly for digestive comfort. However, it should not substitute standard medical therapy for cirrhosis. Always work with your healthcare practitioner to build a thorough treatment plan, including lifestyle adjustments and any required medical procedures.

Slippery Elm Bark

Slippery elm bark (Ulmus rubra) is an herbal treatment recognized for its calming and demulcent characteristics, which may help reduce stomach pain and improve overall gastrointestinal health. While it may not directly cure cirrhosis, it may be used to alleviate some of the symptoms associated with liver diseases. Here's how to prepare and utilize slippery elm bark for cirrhosis health:

Slippery Elm Bark Tea:

Ingredients:
- Dried slippery elm bark (readily accessible at health food shops or online)
- Cold water

Directions:
1. Measure roughly 1-2 tablespoons of dried slippery elm bark per cup of cool water.

2. Gradually add the slippery elm bark to the cold water while stirring frequently to avoid lumps from forming.

3. Let the mixture rest for approximately 5-10 minutes, enabling it to thicken.

4. Drink the slippery elm bark tea while it's still warm.

5. **Frequency:** You may sip slippery elm bark tea up to 2-3 times daily or as required for digestive ease.

Considerations:
- **Visit a Healthcare practitioner:** Before utilizing slippery elm bark for cirrhosis or any other health problem, visit your healthcare practitioner, particularly if you have liver disorders or are taking

drugs. They can advise and verify it is safe and suitable for your unique requirements.

- **Monitor Progress:** Pay attention to how your body reacts to slippery elm bark. Slippery elm is typically safe for most individuals when ingested in modest doses. Some people may have allergies or sensitivities.

- **Safety:** Slippery elm is normally well-tolerated, but it's vital to utilize it in line with suggested doses. Excessive use may lead to possible adverse effects or interactions with drugs.

- **Variety:** You may change the thickness of the tea by adjusting the quantity of slippery elm bark used. If you like a thicker consistency, add more bark; for a thinner tea, use less.

Fennel Seeds

Fennel seeds (Foeniculum vulgare) are commonly used for their possible digestive advantages, including relieving digestive pain and improving healthy digestion. While they may not directly cure cirrhosis, fennel seeds may help control some digestive symptoms linked with liver problems. Here's how to prepare and utilize fennel seeds for cirrhosis health:

Fennel Seed Tea:

Ingredients:

- Fennel seeds (1-2 tablespoons)
- Hot water Honey (optional)

Directions:

1. Measure roughly 1-2 tablespoons of fennel seeds per cup of hot water.

2. Boil water over the fennel seeds in a teapot or cup.

3. Cover the container and let it soak for approximately 5-10 minutes.

4. If desired, add honey for taste.

5. Drink the fennel seed tea while it's still warm.

6. **Frequency:** You may eat fennel seed tea up to 2-3 times daily or as required for digestive relief.

Fennel Seed Chewing:

Ingredients:

- Whole fennel seeds

Directions:

1. Chew on a small handful (approximately 1-2 tablespoons) of whole fennel seeds after a meal.

2. You may also keep a small jar of fennel seeds with you for comfortable chewing throughout the day.

3. **Frequency:** Chew fennel seeds as required, particularly after meals or when you suffer stomach pain.

Considerations:

- **Visit a Healthcare practitioner:** Before using fennel seeds for cirrhosis or any other health problem, visit your healthcare practitioner, particularly if you have liver disorders or are taking drugs. They can advise and verify it is safe and suitable for your unique requirements.

- **Monitor Progress:** Pay attention to how your body reacts to fennel seeds. Fennel seeds are typically safe for most individuals when ingested in modest doses. Some people may have allergies or sensitivities.

- **Safety:** Fennel seeds are generally well-tolerated, but use them in moderation. Excessive use may lead to possible adverse effects or interactions with drugs.

Fennel seeds may be a savory and relaxing addition to your diet, especially if you have stomach distress. However, they should not substitute traditional medical therapy for cirrhosis.

CHAPTER SIX

Herbs to Reduce Inflammation

Licorice Root

Licorice root (Glycyrrhiza glabra) is a plant noted for its potential health advantages, including anti-inflammatory and antioxidant qualities. It may be explored in situations of cirrhosis to promote liver health and control some of the symptoms associated with liver problems. However, licorice root should be taken carefully since it contains chemicals that might influence blood pressure and interact with some drugs. Here's how to prepare and utilize licorice root for cirrhosis health:

Licorice Root Tea:

Ingredients:
- Dried licorice root (readily accessible at health food shops or online)
- Hot water Honey (optional)

Directions:
1. Measure roughly 1-2 tablespoons of dried licorice root per cup of boiling water.

2. Boil water over the dried licorice root in a teapot or cup.

3. Cover the container and let it soak for approximately 5-10 minutes.

4. If desired, add honey for taste.

5. Drink the licorice root tea while it's still warm.

6. **Frequency:** You may eat licorice root tea up to 2-3 times a day, but it's vital to be careful about the length and amount of licorice root consumed due to possible adverse effects.

Considerations:

- **Visit a Healthcare practitioner:** Before using licorice root for cirrhosis health or any other health problem, visit your healthcare practitioner, particularly if you have liver disorders or are taking drugs. Licorice root may alter blood pressure and may interfere with some medicines.

- **Monitor Progress:** Pay attention to how your body reacts to licorice root. Licorice root should be taken in moderation and for short durations to minimize adverse effects.

- **Safety:** Licorice root should not be taken by persons with high blood pressure, heart disorders, or renal difficulties since it may aggravate these diseases. It may also induce fluid retention and potassium loss, leading to imbalances.

- **Duration of Use:** Due to possible adverse effects, licorice root should be taken for brief durations only, often not exceeding a few weeks at a time.

Licorice root may be a beneficial addition to your diet to maintain liver health in instances of cirrhosis. Still, it should be taken with caution and under the advice of a healthcare expert. Always emphasize safety and work with your healthcare practitioner to build a thorough treatment plan, including lifestyle adjustments and any required medical procedures.

Boswellia

Boswellia, often known as Indian frankincense, is an herbal treatment produced from the resin of the Boswellia tree. It's recognized for its possible anti-inflammatory and anti-oxidative qualities. While it may not directly cure cirrhosis, it may help regulate inflammation and promote overall liver function. Here's how to make and utilize Boswellia for cirrhosis health:

Boswellia Capsules or Supplements:

Ingredients:

- Boswellia capsules or supplements (available at health food shops or online)

- Water

Directions:
1. Follow the prescribed dose guidelines on the product label or as your healthcare practitioner suggests.
2. Take the Boswellia pills or supplements with a glass of water or as advised.
3. **Frequency:** Follow the prescribed dose on the product label or your healthcare provider's recommendations.

Considerations:
- **Visit a Healthcare practitioner:** Before taking Boswellia for cirrhosis or any other health problem, visit your healthcare practitioner. They may examine your unique health status, give recommendations on doses, and verify that there are no contraindications or conflicts with drugs you may be taking.

- **Assess Progress:** Regularly evaluate your liver function and general health while taking Boswellia. Discuss any changes in your condition with your healthcare professional.

- **Safety:** Boswellia is usually considered safe for most individuals when used on dietary levels or as a healthcare practitioner suggests. However, some people may develop adverse effects, such as stomach difficulties or allergic responses.

- **Quality Products:** Guarantee you are utilizing high-quality Boswellia supplements from reliable suppliers to guarantee purity and efficacy.

Boswellia might be regarded as a part of a comprehensive strategy for maintaining liver health in instances of cirrhosis. However, it should not replace traditional medical therapy and should be taken with prescription drugs and medical supervision. Always prioritize safety and cooperate with your healthcare physician to build a complete treatment plan.

Cat's Claw

Cat's claw (Uncaria tomentosa) is a herb renowned for its possible anti-inflammatory and immune-boosting qualities. While it may not directly cure cirrhosis, some individuals use a cat's claw to promote general liver function and reduce inflammation. Here's how to prepare and utilize cat's claw for cirrhosis health:

Cat's Claw Tea:

Ingredients:
- Dried cat's claw bark or root (readily accessible at health food shops or online)
- Hot water

Directions:
1. Measure roughly 1-2 tablespoons of dried cat's claw bark or root per cup of boiling water.

2. Boil water over the dried cat's paw in a teapot or cup.

3. Cover the container and let it soak for approximately 10-15 minutes.

4. Strain the tea to remove the cat's claw bits.

5. You may add honey or lemon for taste if preferred.

6. Drink the cat's paw tea while it's still warm.

7. **Frequency:** You may eat cat's claw tea up to 2-3 times a day or as a healthcare practitioner prescribes.

Cat's Claw Capsules or Supplements:

Ingredients:
- Cat's claw pills or supplements (available at health food shops or online)
- Water

Directions:
1. Follow the prescribed dose guidelines on the product label or as your healthcare practitioner suggests.
2. Take the cat's claw capsules or supplements with a glass of water or as advised.

3. **Frequency:** Follow the prescribed dose on the product label or your healthcare provider's recommendations.

Considerations:

- **Visit a Healthcare practitioner:** Before using a cat's claw for cirrhosis or any other health problem, visit your healthcare practitioner. They may examine your unique health status, give recommendations on doses, and verify that there are no contraindications or conflicts with drugs you may be taking.

- **Assess Progress:** Regularly assess your liver function and general health using a cat's claw. Discuss any changes in your condition with your healthcare professional.

- **Safety:** Cat's claw is usually considered safe for most individuals when ingested at dietary levels or as a healthcare practitioner prescribes. However, some people may develop adverse effects, such as stomach difficulties or allergic responses.

- **Quality Products:** Guarantee you are utilizing high-quality cat's claw supplements from reliable suppliers to guarantee purity and efficacy.

Cat's claw might be regarded as part of a comprehensive strategy to promote liver health in instances of cirrhosis. However, it should not replace traditional medical therapy and should be taken with prescription drugs and medical supervision. Always prioritize safety and cooperate with your healthcare physician to build a complete treatment plan.

Holy Basil

Holy basil, commonly known as Tulsi (Ocimum sanctum or Ocimum tenuiflorum), is a plant noted for its possible health benefits, including anti-inflammatory and antioxidant qualities. While it may not directly cure cirrhosis, holy basil may promote general liver function and decrease inflammation. Here's how to make and utilize holy basil for cirrhosis health:

Holy Basil Tea:

Ingredients:
- Fresh holy basil leaves (a handful) or dried holy basil leaves (readily accessible at health food shops or online)
- Hot water
- Honey (optional)

Directions:
1. If using fresh holy basil leaves, wash and cut them.

2. Measure around 1-2 tablespoons per cup of hot water using dried holy basil leaves.

3. In a teapot or cup, boil water over the fresh or dried holy basil leaves.

4. Cover the container and let it soak for approximately 5-10 minutes.

5. If desired, add honey for taste.

6. Drink the holy basil tea while it's still warm.

7. **Frequency:** You may sip holy basil tea up to 2-3 times a day or as required for its possible advantages.

Considerations:

- **Visit a Healthcare practitioner:** Before using holy basil for cirrhosis or any other health problem, visit your healthcare practitioner, particularly if you have liver disorders or are taking drugs. They can advise and verify it is safe and suitable for your unique requirements.

- **Monitor Progress:** Pay attention to how your body reacts to holy basil. Holy basil is typically safe for most individuals when ingested in modest doses. Some people may have allergies or sensitivities.

- **Safety:** Holy basil is usually well-tolerated, but consume it in moderation. Excessive intake may lead to possible adverse effects.

- **Variety:** You may change the intensity of your holy basil tea by adjusting the number of holy basil leaves used or the steeping duration.

Holy basil may be a tasty and relaxing addition to your diet and may give advantages for liver health in cirrhosis. However, it should not replace traditional medical therapy and should be taken with prescription drugs and medical supervision. Always prioritize safety and cooperate with your healthcare physician to build a complete treatment plan.

CHAPTER SEVEN

Herbal Remedies for Managing Symptoms

Ascites and Edema

Ascites and edema are typical consequences of cirrhosis, a late stage of scarring (fibrosis) of the liver produced by long-term liver damage. These disorders develop due to the liver's reduced capacity to handle fluids and proteins, resulting in fluid retention in the abdomen (ascites) and swelling in other body regions (edema). Here's a deeper look at each condition:

1. Ascites:

What Is Ascites?

Ascites are the buildup of excess fluid in the abdominal cavity. It is a frequent consequence of cirrhosis and may also arise from other illnesses, such as heart failure or some malignancies.

1. **Causes:** In cirrhosis, the damaged liver fails to generate enough albumin, a protein crucial for maintaining fluid balance. Consequently, fluid escapes from blood vessels into the abdominal cavity, creating ascites.

2. **Symptoms:** Ascites may lead to stomach swelling and pain. In extreme situations, it may cause breathing difficulties and strain internal organs.

3. **Management:** Managing ascites often entails dietary salt restriction, diuretic drugs (to remove excess fluid), paracentesis (a technique to drain fluid from the belly), and resolving the underlying liver illness.

2. Edema:

What Is Edema?

Edema is the swelling of bodily tissues, frequently visible in the ankles, feet, legs, and occasionally in the hands and face. It happens when extra fluid collects in the body's tissues.

1. **Causes:** Edema in cirrhosis is generally due to a combination of reasons, including reduced albumin synthesis by the liver, increased pressure in blood vessels, and fluid retention.

2. **Symptoms:** Edema leads to noticeable swelling and might cause pain. In extreme situations, it may limit movement and lead to consequences, including skin infections.

3. **Care:** The care of edema entails many of the same methods used for ascites, such as sodium

restriction, diuretics, and treating the underlying liver illness.

Engaging closely with a healthcare practitioner and following their suggestions for treating ascites and edema in cirrhosis is crucial. These illnesses may become severe and lead to problems if left untreated. In severe cirrhosis, liver transplantation may be explored as a therapy option. Additionally, patients with cirrhosis should avoid alcohol totally and take precautions to prevent additional liver damage.

Lifestyle adjustments, dietary changes, and medicines may help manage these symptoms. Still, they should always be evaluated by a healthcare professional to verify they are suitable for the individual's condition and the underlying liver illness.

Jaundice

Jaundice is a medical disorder marked by the yellowing of the skin, mucous membranes, and the whites of the eyes. It happens when there is an excess of bilirubin in the blood, a yellow pigment generated during the breakdown of red blood cells. Jaundice may indicate numerous underlying medical disorders, including liver disease, and it can present in persons with cirrhosis.

1. **Causes:** Jaundice may be caused by several reasons, including liver illnesses such as cirrhosis, hepatitis, alcoholic liver disease, and bile duct blockages. It may also arise from hemolytic anemia (excessive breakdown of red blood cells), some drugs, and hereditary disorders.

2. **Symptoms:** The primary sign of jaundice is the yellowing of the skin, eyes, and mucous membranes. Other symptoms may include dark urine, pale feces, weariness, stomach discomfort, itching (pruritus), and changes in appetite.

3. **Diagnosis:** A healthcare professional will diagnose jaundice using a physical examination, medical history, and blood tests to assess bilirubin levels. Additional testing, such as imaging investigations or liver function tests, may be undertaken to discover the underlying reason.

4. **Treatment:** Treatment for jaundice relies on treating the underlying cause. In cirrhosis-related jaundice, the main objective is to control and treat the cirrhosis itself. This may require dietary adjustments, medicine to control symptoms and problems, and, in advanced situations, liver transplantation.

5. **Consequences:** Untreated jaundice or the underlying disorders producing jaundice may lead to significant results, including liver failure, renal

issues, and encephalopathy (a brain abnormality linked with liver disease).

6. **Prevention:** Preventing jaundice frequently entails treating the underlying causes. Lifestyle adjustments, such as avoiding excessive alcohol intake and practicing safe sex to prevent hepatitis infection, may help minimize the incidence of liver-related jaundice.

Jaundice may be an indication of a dangerous medical problem, and anybody suffering signs of jaundice should seek medical assistance soon. Early identification and treatment of the underlying cause are critical for treating the disease and avoiding consequences. Individuals with cirrhosis should work closely with their healthcare practitioner to monitor and manage their liver function to prevent or resolve jaundice and its accompanying problems.

Fatigue and Weakness

Fatigue and weakness are frequent symptoms reported by patients with cirrhosis and may significantly influence their quality of life. These symptoms may have numerous origins and may be connected to the underlying liver disease and its consequences. Here are some crucial aspects to grasp about weariness and weakness in cirrhosis:

Causes of Fatigue and Weakness:

1. **Liver Dysfunction:** In cirrhosis, the liver's capacity to execute vital processes, such as filtering toxins and making proteins, is diminished. This may lead to an accumulation of waste products in the body, resulting in weariness.
2. **Anemia:** Cirrhosis may lead to a reduction in red blood cell synthesis, leading to anemia. Anemia may produce weariness and weakness due to diminished blood oxygen-carrying capacity.
3. **Nutritional Deficiencies:** Poor appetite, malabsorption of nutrients, and poor food intake may contribute to dietary deficiencies, resulting in weakness and weariness.
4. **Infection:** Cirrhosis may impair the immune system, making persons more prone to infections, which can induce weariness.
5. **Fluid Retention:** Conditions like ascites (abdominal fluid buildup) and edema (swelling) may contribute to pain and weariness.
6. **Medications:** Medications that address cirrhosis-related symptoms or consequences may have adverse effects that lead to tiredness.

Symptoms:

- Fatigue is a constant sense of fatigue, exhaustion, or lack of energy.

- Weakness refers to a diminished physical or muscular strength, which might impede everyday tasks.

Management of weariness and weakness in cirrhosis entails treating the underlying causes:
- They are treating the underlying liver disease, such as cirrhosis or hepatitis.
- Managing problems including ascites, edema, or hepatic encephalopathy.
- She was addressing nutritional inadequacies via dietary adjustments and supplementation.
- We are monitoring and controlling anemia with the support of a healthcare practitioner.
- In certain situations, physical activity and exercise suited to an individual's condition might assist in enhancing muscular strength and energy levels.

- A balanced and healthy diet, high in protein and essential vitamins and minerals, may help overcome weakness and weariness.
- Consult with a trained nutritionist for individualized dietary suggestions.

Lifestyle:

- Adequate rest and sleep are vital for controlling tiredness. Establish a consistent sleep schedule and emphasize quality sleep.
- Avoid excessive alcohol intake since it might increase liver damage and exhaustion.
- Manage stress with relaxation methods, such as deep breathing and meditation.

Medication Management:

- Review and modify medicines with a healthcare professional to reduce adverse effects related to tiredness.

Monitoring:

- Regular medical checks and monitoring of liver function, blood counts, and nutritional status are critical for controlling lethargy and weakness in cirrhosis.

Patients with cirrhosis must work closely with their healthcare physician to identify and treat the reasons for weariness and weakness. Tailored treatment programs, lifestyle improvements, and appropriate medical treatments may increase energy levels and general well-being.

Itchy Skin

Itchy skin, medically known as pruritus, maybe a distressing symptom experienced by patients with cirrhosis. Itchy skin in cirrhosis may come from several sources, including liver dysfunction and the consequences of the illness. Here's what you should know about itching skin and cirrhosis:

Causes of Itchy Skin in Cirrhosis:

1. **Bile Duct blockage:** In cirrhosis, damage to the liver may lead to bile duct blockage or dysfunction. This might result in the buildup of bile salts in the circulation, which can cause itching.

2. **Accumulation of Toxins:** The liver performs a critical function in detoxifying the body. When the liver is damaged, toxins may build in the circulation, perhaps leading to itching.

3. **Hepatic Encephalopathy:** Cirrhosis-related hepatic encephalopathy, a disorder characterized by brain dysfunction, may induce behavioral abnormalities and itching.

4. **Dry Skin:** Individuals with cirrhosis may also develop dry skin, aggravated by factors like dehydration or drugs.

5. **Complications:** Conditions linked with cirrhosis, such as ascites (abdominal fluid buildup) and edema (swelling), may add to skin pain and itching.

Treating the Underlying Cause: Addressing the underlying liver illness and its repercussions is critical. Managing cirrhosis with lifestyle modifications, drugs, and, in rare instances, liver transplantation may help ease symptoms.

- **Drugs:** In rare circumstances, healthcare practitioners may prescribe medications to ease itching. Antihistamines or bile acid-binding medicines may alleviate itching associated with liver disease.

- **Skin Care:** Proper skin care is vital for controlling itching:

- ✓ Use mild, fragrance-free moisturizers to keep the skin nourished.
- ✓ Avoid hot showers and use lukewarm water for bathing.
- ✓ Choose mild, hypoallergenic soaps and detergents.
- ✓ Pat the skin dry after showering; avoid rubbing aggressively.
- ✓ Maintain proper cleanliness to avoid infections since scratching may lead to skin issues.

- **Cooling Measures:** Applying cold compresses to irritated regions might give temporary relief.

- **Avoid Scratching:** While tough, avoid scratching the itching skin since it may lead to skin damage and infections. Keep nails short to prevent the danger of tearing the skin when scratching.

- **Diet and Nutrition:** Maintain a well-balanced diet and remain hydrated to improve overall skin health.

- **Stress Management:** Stress may increase itching. Practicing relaxation methods such as deep breathing or meditation may assist.

- **Visit a Healthcare practitioner:** If itching is severe or continues after self-care methods, visit a healthcare practitioner for a comprehensive examination and further treatment options.

Discuss any symptoms you feel, including itching, with your healthcare professional since it might indicate underlying concerns. They can assist in discovering the origin of the itching and give suitable counseling and therapy customized to your unique situation.

CHAPTER EIGHT

Incorporating Herbal Remedies into Your Routine

Dosage & Administration

Incorporating herbal medicines into your regimen needs careful consideration of the exact herbs you plan to utilize, their suggested doses, and administration techniques. Please note that herbal treatments should be taken carefully and under the advice of a healthcare expert, particularly if you have underlying medical concerns or are taking drugs. Here are some broad tips for adding herbal treatments to your routine:

1. Consult a Healthcare Provider:

- Before taking any herbal medicine, ask your healthcare professional to confirm it's safe and acceptable for your unique health requirements and any interactions with pharmaceuticals.

2. Choose High-Quality Herbs:

- Select trusted sources for acquiring herbs to assure their purity and efficacy.

3. Determine Dosage:

- The optimal dose of herbal medicines might vary greatly depending on the plant and the particular health condition you're treating.
- Dosages are typically indicated on the product label; however, speaking with a herbalist or naturopathic doctor may assist in identifying the proper amount for your requirements.

4. Start with Low Doses:

- If you're new to a particular herbal medicine, start with a lesser dosage and evaluate your body's reaction before increasing it.
- Gradually titrate the dose to obtain the desired effect, if required.

5. Administration Methods:

- Herbal medicines may be delivered in numerous forms, including teas, tinctures, capsules, pills, and topical treatments (creams or ointments).
- The choice of administration technique may depend on the plant and your inclination.

6. Consistency is Key:

- To experience the potential advantages of herbal treatments, utilizing them regularly over time is generally required.

- Follow the suggested dose regimen, and be patient, since it may take weeks or even months to see effects in some circumstances.

7. Monitor for Adverse Effects:

- Pay careful attention to how your body reacts to herbal medicines.
- Be aware of any possible adverse effects, allergic reactions, or interactions with any drugs you may be taking.
- If you encounter any harmful effects, cease usage and inform your healthcare professional.

8. Keep Records:

- Maintain a record of your herbal treatments, including doses and administration methods.
- This might help you monitor their efficacy and exchange information with your healthcare professional.

9. Adjust as Needed:

- Periodically check the efficiency of herbal treatments in resolving your health difficulties.
- Be open to changing your herbal regimen if required.

Remember that herbal medicines do not replace regular medical therapy, particularly for severe diseases like cirrhosis. Always work with your healthcare physician to build a complete treatment plan that integrates traditional medical procedures with any herbal medicines you wish to use. Your healthcare practitioner can advise on safety, effectiveness, and possible interactions with your existing drugs or therapies.

Creating Herbal Formulas

Creating herbal formulations for cirrhosis needs careful study of the individual plants, their potential benefits, and their interactions. Engaging closely with a skilled healthcare professional, such as a naturopathic doctor or herbalist, who can adapt a herbal formula to your unique requirements and evaluate its success is crucial. Here are some herbs widely regarded for cirrhosis and how they may be mixed into a formula:

Note: Always contact a healthcare physician before taking herbal medicines, particularly if you have cirrhosis or other underlying medical issues.

1. Milk Thistle (Silybum marianum):
   - Milk thistle is one of the most well-known herbs for liver health and is regularly used in herbal recipes for cirrhosis.
   - It may help protect and maintain the liver by lowering inflammation and oxidative damage.

2. Dandelion Root (Taraxacum officinale):
   - Dandelion root is considered to boost liver function and promote good digestion.

- It might be added to relieve stomach issues frequently linked with cirrhosis.

3. Turmeric (Curcuma longa):
- Turmeric includes curcumin, recognized for its anti-inflammatory and antioxidant effects.
- It may help minimize liver inflammation and enhance overall liver health.

4. Schisandra Berry (Schisandra chinensis):
- Schisandra is an adaptogenic plant that may help the liver adapt to stress and prevent oxidative damage.
- It's included for its possible protective effects on the liver.

5. Burdock Root (Arctium lappa):
- Burdock root is known to help liver detoxification and enhance overall liver function.
- It may be added for its putative detoxifying qualities.

6. Artichoke Leaf (Cynara scolymus):
- Artichoke leaf boosts bile synthesis and enhances liver and gallbladder function.
- It may assist in improving digestion and alleviating stomach pain.

7. Licorice Root (Glycyrrhiza glabra):
- Licorice root may be incorporated for its possible anti-inflammatory and calming effects on the digestive tract.

- It should be taken with care owing to its possible influence on blood pressure.

8. Yellow Dock (Rumex crispus):

- Yellow dock may boost liver function and aid with digestive disorders.
- It's included for its possible effects on overall digestion.

Sample Herbal Formula for Cirrhosis

A trained healthcare physician may build a personalized herbal formula depending on your unique requirements and the severity of your cirrhosis. Here's a basic example:

- **Milk Thistle (Silybum marianum):** 300 mg
- **Dandelion Root (Taraxacum officinale):** 200 mg
- **Turmeric (Curcuma longa):** 150 mg
- **Schisandra Berry (Schisandra chinensis):** 100 mg
- **Burdock Root (Arctium lappa):** 100 mg
- **Artichoke Leaf (Cynara scolymus):** 100 mg

Dosages and ratios might vary based on the individual's condition and the exact herbal extracts or forms employed (e.g., capsules, tinctures, teas). It's vital to have a healthcare expert analyze your situation, do any required tests, and monitor your progress while utilizing the herbal mixture.

This is a typical example, and the exact formula should be changed depending on your unique health requirements, the degree of cirrhosis, and any possible interactions with drugs or other therapies you may be undergoing. Always emphasize safety and work closely with a certified healthcare physician while utilizing herbal formulations for cirrhosis.

Monitoring Progress

When introducing herbal medicines into your regimen, you must evaluate your progress carefully to ensure they are helpful and safe for your unique requirements. Here are some ways to help you track your success while utilizing herbal remedies:

1. Consult a Healthcare Provider:

- Before commencing any herbal cure, seek a trained healthcare professional informed about herbal medicine. They can assist you in identifying the proper herbs, doses, and formulations depending on your health situation.

2. Keep a Health Journal:

- Maintain a health diary to chronicle your symptoms, improvements, and any changes you find while utilizing herbal medicines.
- Record each dose's date, time, and specifics, including the herb, Dosage, and any adverse effects or improvements.

3. Monitor Symptoms:

- Pay special attention to the symptoms or health conditions you address with herbal medicines.
- Note any changes, improvements, or worsening of symptoms over time.

4. Regular Follow-Up with a Healthcare Provider:

- Schedule frequent follow-up sessions with your healthcare practitioner to review your progress.
- Share the information from your health diary to offer a complete summary of your experience with herbal therapies.

5. Laboratory Tests:

- In rare situations, your healthcare physician may request laboratory testing to monitor your condition and the effect of herbal medicines.
- These tests may include liver function tests, blood counts, or other pertinent indicators dependent on your health concerns.

6. Be Patient:

- Herbal medicines may take a while to show their benefits. Some changes may be slow, so be patient and allow the treatments time to work.
- Follow the prescribed doses and directions supplied by your healthcare professional or herbalist.

7. Adjustments as Needed:

- Share these changes with your healthcare physician if you discover significant improvements or harmful effects.
- Adjustments to the herbal medicine regimen may be required, depending on your success.

8. Monitor for Side Effects:

- Watch for any side effects or inadequate responses to the herbal therapies.
- Common side effects may include stomach difficulties, allergic reactions, or interactions with other drugs.

9. Document Dietary and Lifestyle Changes:

- Document these changes in your health diary if you're making dietary or lifestyle modifications with herbal medicines.
- This information may assist in discovering possible contributions to your development.

10. Stay Informed:

- Continue educating yourself on your herbs and their possible advantages or hazards.
- Stay updated about new research or advances connected to herbal medicines and your health condition.

-    If you suffer any unpleasant effects or your condition worsens, seek quick counsel from your healthcare physician or herbalist.

Combining Herbs with Lifestyle Changes

Combining herbal medicines with lifestyle modifications may be an effective method for enhancing liver health and controlling cirrhosis. Lifestyle adjustments may assist in supporting the liver and boost the potential effects of herbal medicines. Here are some lifestyle modifications to consider when including herbs in your cirrhosis health plan:

1. Dietary Changes:
-    **Reduce Sodium Intake:** Limit salt intake to control fluid retention, particularly if you have ascites or edema.
-    **Choose a Balanced Diet:** Consume a diet rich in fruits, vegetables, whole grains, lean proteins, and healthy fats.
-    **Moderate Protein Intake:** Aim for average protein intake to maintain muscle mass and support liver function.

2. Hydration:
-    **Stay Hydrated:** Drink an appropriate quantity of water to avoid dehydration, but observe any fluid limitations prescribed by your healthcare practitioner.

3. Alcohol Avoidance:

- **Complete Abstinence:** Avoid alcohol, which might aggravate liver damage and cirrhosis.

4. Medication Management:

- Consult with a Healthcare Provider: Discuss any drugs and supplements you take with your healthcare physician to prevent possible interactions or liver damage.

5. Weight Management:

- Achieve and Maintain a Healthy Weight: If overweight, consult a healthcare physician to design a weight management strategy to lessen stress on the liver.

6. Physical Activity:

- Frequent Exercise: Engage in regular, moderate exercise, as advised by your healthcare physician, to promote general health and well-being.

7. Stress Reduction:

- Stress Management: Practice stress-reduction strategies such as deep breathing, meditation, yoga, or mindfulness to promote general health.

8. Avoid Hepatitis Risk:

- Safe Practices: Take care to prevent hepatitis infection by practicing safe sex and avoiding sharing needles or personal things that may transfer the virus.

9. Monitoring and Follow-Up:

- Regular Checkups: Maintain regular medical and follow-up consultations with your healthcare practitioner to monitor your liver function and general health.

10. Herbal Remedies:

- **Consultation:** Work with a certified healthcare physician or herbalist to pick suitable herbs and establish a customized regimen based on your health requirements and objectives.
- **Consistency:** Take herbal treatments regularly, following the stated doses and directions.

11. Sleep Hygiene:

- Healthy Sleep Habits: Establish a regular sleep regimen and emphasize quality sleep for general well-being.

12. Avoid Toxins:

- Limit Exposure: Minimize exposure to environmental toxins, such as chemicals and pollution, to lessen the liver's burden.

13. Social Support:

- Engage in a Supportive Network: Seek emotional assistance from friends, family, or support groups to help deal with the problems of managing cirrhosis.

- Stay educated: Educate yourself about cirrhosis, its care, and its consequences to become an educated champion for your health.

Remember that cirrhosis is a complicated illness, and individual requirements might differ. Your healthcare professional should be vital in coaching you through these lifestyle modifications and implementing herbal therapies into your cirrhosis health plan. They can help you establish a thorough and tailored strategy for treating your disease efficiently.